My Mediterranean
Cookbook

Tasty And Affordable Mediterranean Recipes To
Start Your Day With The Right Foot

Dan Peterson

TABLE OF CONTENT

Papaya, Jicama, and Peas Rice Bowl

Preparation time: 15 minutes

Cooking time: 45 minutes

Servings: 4

INGREDIENTS:

Sauce:
Juice of ¼ lemon
2 teaspoons chopped fresh basil
1 tablespoon raw honey
1 tablespoon extra-virgin olive oil
Sea salt, to taste
Rice:
1½ cups wild rice
2 papayas, peeled, seeded, and diced
1 jicama, peeled and shredded
1 cup snow peas, julienned
2 cups shredded cabbage
1 scallion, white and green parts, chopped

DIRECTIONS:

Combine the ingredients for the sauce in a bowl. Stir to mix well. Set aside until ready to use. Pour the wild rice in a saucepan, then pour in enough water to cover. Bring to a boil.

Reduce the heat to low, then simmer for 45 minutes or until the wild rice is soft and plump. Drain and transfer to a large serving bowl.

Top the rice with papayas, jicama, peas, cabbage, and scallion. Pour the sauce over and stir to

mix well before serving.
NUTRITION: Calories: 446 Fat: 7.9g Protein: 13.1g
Carbs: 85.8g

Wild Rice, Celery, and Cauliflower Pilaf

Preparation time: 15 minutes

Cooking time: 45 minutes

Servings: 4

INGREDIENTS:

  1 tablespoon olive oil, plus more for greasing the baking dish
  1 cup wild rice
  2 cups low-sodium chicken broth
  1 sweet onion, chopped
  2 stalks celery, chopped
  1 teaspoon minced garlic
  2 carrots, peeled, halved lengthwise, and sliced
  ½ cauliflower head, cut into small florets
  1 teaspoon chopped fresh thyme
  Sea salt, to taste

DIRECTIONS:

  Preheat the oven to 350ºF (180ºC). Line a baking sheet with parchment paper and grease with olive oil.

  Put the wild rice in a saucepan, then pour in the chicken broth. Bring to a boil. Reduce the heat to low and simmer for 30 minutes or until the rice is plump.

  Meanwhile, heat the remaining olive oil in an oven-proof skillet over medium-high heat until shimmering.

Add the onion, celery, and garlic to the skillet and sauté for 3 minutes or until the onion is translucent.

Add the carrots and cauliflower to the skillet and sauté for 5 minutes. Turn off the heat and set aside.

Pour the cooked rice in the skillet with the vegetables. Sprinkle with thyme and salt. Set the skillet in the preheated oven and bake for 15 minutes or until the vegetables are soft. Serve immediately.

NUTRITION: Calories: 214 Fat: 3.9g Protein: 7.2g Carbs: 37.9g

Minestrone Chickpeas and Macaroni Casserole

Preparation time : 15 minutes
Cooking time: 7 hours & 25 minutes

Servings: 5

INGREDIENTS:

- 1 (15-ounce / 425-g) can chickpeas, drained and rinsed
- 1 (28-ounce / 794-g) can diced tomatoes, with the juice
- 1 (6-ounce / 170-g) can no-salt-added tomato paste
- 3 medium carrots, sliced
- 3 cloves garlic, minced
- 1 medium yellow onion, chopped
- 1 cup low-sodium vegetable soup
- ½ teaspoon dried rosemary
- 1 teaspoon dried oregano
- 2 teaspoons maple syrup
- ½ teaspoon sea salt
- ¼ teaspoon ground black pepper
- ½ pound (227-g) fresh green beans, trimmed and cut into bite-size pieces
- 1 cup macaroni pasta
- 2 ounces (57 g) Parmesan cheese, grated

DIRECTIONS:

Except for the green beans, pasta, and Parmesan cheese, combine all the ingredients in the slow cooker and stir to mix well. Put the slow cooker lid on and cook on low for 7 hours.

Fold in the pasta and green beans. Put the lid on and cook on high for 20 minutes or until the vegetable are soft and the pasta is al dente.

Pour them in a large serving bowl and spread with Parmesan cheese before serving.

NUTRITION: Calories: 349 Fat: 6.7g Protein: 16.5g Carbs: 59.9g

Small Pasta and Beans Pot

Preparation time: 15 minutes

Cooking time: 15 minutes

Servings: 2-4

INGREDIENTS:
- 1 pound (454 g) small whole wheat pasta
- 1 (14.5-ounce / 411-g) can diced tomatoes, juice reserved
- 1 (15-ounce / 425-g) can cannellini beans, drained and rinsed
- 2 tablespoons no-salt-added tomato paste
- 1 red or yellow bell pepper, chopped
- 1 yellow onion, chopped
- 1 tablespoon Italian seasoning mix
- 3 garlic cloves, minced
- ¼ teaspoon crushed red pepper flakes, optional
- 1 tablespoon extra-virgin olive oil
- 5 cups water
- 1 bunch kale, stemmed and chopped
- ½ cup pitted Kalamata olives, chopped
- 1 cup sliced basil

DIRECTIONS:
- Except for the kale, olives, and basil, combine all the ingredients in a pot. Stir to mix well. Bring to a boil over high heat. Stir constantly.
- Reduce the heat to medium high and add the kale. Cook for 10 minutes or until the pasta is al dente. Stir constantly. Transfer all of them on a large plate and serve with olives and basil on

top.
NUTRITION: Calories: 357 Fat: 7.6g Protein: 18.2g
Carbs: 64.5g

Italian Baked Beans

Preparation time: 5 minutes

Cooking time: 15 minutes

Servings: 6

INGREDIENTS:

 2 teaspoons extra-virgin olive oil
 ½ cup minced onion (about ¼ onion)
 1 (12-ounce) can low-sodium tomato paste
 ¼ cup red wine vinegar
 2 tablespoons honey
 ¼ teaspoon ground cinnamon
 ½ cup water
 2 (15-ounce) cans cannellini or great northern beans, undrained

DIRECTIONS:

In a medium saucepan over medium heat, heat the oil. Add the onion and cook for 5 minutes, stirring frequently.

Add the tomato paste, vinegar, honey, cinnamon, and water, and mix well. Turn the heat to low. Drain and rinse one can of the beans in a colander and add to the saucepan.

Pour the entire second can of beans (including the liquid) into the saucepan. Let it cook for 10 minutes, stirring occasionally, and serve.

Ingredient tip: Switch up this recipe by making new variations of the homemade ketchup. Instead of the cinnamon, try ¼ teaspoon of smoked paprika and 1 tablespoon of hot sauce.

Serve.
NUTRITION: Calories: 236 Fat: 3g Carbohydrates: 42g
Protein: 10g

Tahini Pine Nuts Toast

Preparation Time: 5 minutes
Cooking Time : 0 minutes

Servings: 2

INGREDIENTS:
  2 whole-wheat bread slices, toasted
  1 tsp. water
  1 tbsp. tahini paste
  2 tsps. feta cheese, crumbled
  Juice of ½ lemon
  2 tsps. pine nuts
  A pinch of black pepper

DIRECTIONS:
  In a bowl, mix the tahini with the water and the lemon juice, whisk well, and spread over the toasted bread slices. Top each serving with the remaining ingredients and serve for breakfast.
NUTRITION: Calories 142 Fat: 7.6g Carbs: 13.7g
Protein: 5.8g

Feta - Avocado & Mashed Chickpea Toast

Preparation Time: 10 minutes
Cooking Time : 15 minutes

Servings: 4

INGREDIENTS:

    15 oz. can Chickpeas
    2 oz. - ½ cup Diced feta cheese
    1 Pitted avocado
    Fresh juice:
    2 tsp. Lemon (or 1 tbsp. orange)
    ½ tsp. Black pepper
    2 tsp. Honey
    4 slices Multigrain toast

DIRECTIONS:

    Toast the bread. Drain the chickpeas in a colander. Scoop the avocado flesh into the bowl. Use a large fork/potato masher to mash them until the mix is spreadable.

    Pour in the lemon juice, pepper, and feta. Combine and divide onto the four slices of toast. Drizzle using the honey and serve.

NUTRITION: Calories: 337 Carbs: 43g Fat: 13g Protein: 13g

Feta Frittata

Preparation Time: 15 minutes

Cooking Time: 25 minutes

Servings: 2

INGREDIENTS:
- 1 small clove Garlic
- 1 Green onion
- 2 Large eggs
- ½ cup Egg substitute
- 4 tbsp. Crumbled feta cheese - divided
- 1/3 cup Plum tomato
- 4 thin Avocado slices
- 2 tbsp. Reduced-fat sour cream
- Also Needed: 6-inch skillet

DIRECTIONS:
- Thinly slice/mince the onion, garlic, and tomato. Peel the avocado before slicing. Heat the pan using the medium temperature setting and spritz it with cooking oil.
- Whisk the egg substitute, eggs, and the feta cheese. Add the egg mixture into the pan. Cover and simmer for four to six minutes.
- Sprinkle it using the rest of the feta cheese and tomato. Cover and continue cooking until the eggs are set or about two to three more minutes.
- Wait for about five minutes before cutting it into halves. Serve with the avocado and sour cream.

NUTRITION: Calories: 460 Carbs: 8g Fat: 37g Protein: 24g

Smoked Salmon and Poached Eggs on Toast

Preparation Time: 10 minutes

Cooking Time : 4 minutes

Servings: 4

INGREDIENTS:

2 oz avocado smashed

2 slices of bread toasted

Pinch of kosher salt and cracked black pepper

1/4 tsp freshly squeezed lemon juice

2 eggs see notes, poached

3.5 oz smoked salmon

1 TBSP. thinly sliced scallions

Splash of Kikkoman soy sauce optional

Microgreens are optional

DIRECTIONS:

Take a small bowl and then smash the avocado into it. Then, add the lemon juice and also a pinch of salt into the mixture. Then, mix it well and set aside.

After that, poach the eggs and toast the bread for some time. Once the bread is toasted, you will have to spread the avocado on both slices and after that, add the smoked salmon to each slice.

Thereafter, carefully transfer the poached eggs to the respective toasts. Add a splash of Kikkoman soy sauce and some cracked pepper; then, just garnish with scallions and microgreens.

NUTRITION: Calories: 459 Protein: 31 g Fat: 22 g Carbs: 33 g

Honey Almond Ricotta Spread with Peaches

Preparation Time: 5 minutes

Cooking Time: 8 minutes

Servings: 4

INGREDIENTS:

1/2 cup Fisher Sliced Almonds

1 cup whole milk ricotta

1/4 teaspoon almond extract

zest from an orange, optional

1 teaspoon honey

hearty whole-grain toast

English muffin or bagel

extra Fisher sliced almonds

sliced peaches

extra honey for drizzling

DIRECTIONS:

Cut peaches into a proper shape and then brush them with olive oil. After that, set it aside. Take a bowl; combine the ingredients for the filling. Set aside.

Then just pre-heat grill to medium. Place peaches cut side down onto the greased grill. Close lid cover and then just grill until the peaches have softened, approximately 6-10 minutes, depending on the size of the peaches.

Then you will have to place peach halves onto a serving plate. Put a spoon of about 1 tablespoon of ricotta mixture into the cavity (you are also allowed to use a small scooper).

Sprinkle it with slivered almonds, crushed amaretti cookies, and honey. Decorate with the mint leaves.

NUTRITION: Calories: 187 Protein: 7 g Fat: 9 g Carbs: 18 g

Mediterranean Eggs Cups

Preparation Time: 10 minutes

Cooking Time: 20 minutes

Servings: 8

INGREDIENTS:

1 cup spinach, finely diced

1/2 yellow onion, finely diced

1/2 cup sliced sun-dried tomatoes

4 large basil leaves, finely diced

Pepper and salt to taste

1/3 cup feta cheese crumbles

8 large eggs

1/4 cup milk (any kind)

DIRECTIONS:

Warm the oven to 375°F. Then, roll the dough sheet into a 12x8-inch rectangle. Then, cut in half lengthwise.

After that, you will have to cut each half crosswise into 4 pieces, forming 8 (4x3-inch) pieces dough. Then, press each into the bottom and up sides of the ungreased muffin cup.

Trim dough to keep the dough from touching, if essential. Set aside. Then, you will have to combine the eggs, salt, pepper in the bowl and beat it with a whisk until well mixed. Set aside.

Melt the butter in 12-inch skillet over medium heat until sizzling; add bell peppers. You will have to cook it, stirring occasionally, 2-3 minutes or until crisply tender.

After that, add spinach leaves; continue cooking until spinach is wilted. Then just add egg mixture and prosciutto.

Divide the mixture evenly among prepared muffin cups. Finally, bake it for 14-17 minutes or until the crust is golden brown.

NUTRITION: Calories: 240 Protein: 9 g Fat: 16 g Carbs: 13 g

Low-Carb Baked Eggs with Avocado and Feta

Preparation Time: 10 minutes

Cooking Time: 15 minutes

Servings: 2

INGREDIENTS:

1 avocado

4 eggs

2-3 tbsp. crumbled feta cheese

Nonstick cooking spray

Pepper and salt to taste

DIRECTIONS:

First, you will have to preheat the oven to 400 degrees F. After that, when the oven is on the proper temperature, you will have to put the gratin dishes right on the baking sheet.

Then, leave the dishes to heat in the oven for almost 10 minutes After that process, you need to break the eggs into individual ramekins.

Then, let the avocado and eggs come to room temperature for at least 10 minutes. Then, peel the avocado properly and cut it each half into 6 -8 slices.

You will have to remove the dishes from the oven and spray them with the non-stick spray. Then, you will have to arrange all the sliced avocados in the dishes and tip two eggs into each dish. Sprinkle with feta, add pepper and salt to taste, serve.

NUTRITION: Calories: 280 Protein: 11 g Fat: 23 g Carbs: 10 g

Mediterranean Eggs White Breakfast Sandwich with Roasted Tomatoes

Preparation Time: 15 minutes

Cooking Time: 10 minutes

Servings: 2

INGREDIENTS:

Salt and pepper to taste

¼ cup egg whites

1 teaspoon chopped fresh herbs like rosemary, basil, parsley,

1 whole-grain seeded ciabatta roll

1 teaspoon butter

1-2 slices Muenster cheese

1 tablespoon pesto

About ½ cup roasted tomatoes

10 ounces grape tomatoes

1 tablespoon extra-virgin olive oil

Black pepper and salt to taste

DIRECTIONS:

First, you will have to melt the butter over medium heat in the small nonstick skillet. Then, mix the egg whites with pepper and salt.

Then, sprinkle it with the fresh herbs. After that cook it for almost 3-4 minutes or until the eggs are done, then flip it carefully.

Meanwhile, toast ciabatta bread in the toaster. Place the egg on the bottom half of the sandwich rolls, then top with cheese

Add roasted tomatoes and the top half of roll. To make a roasted tomato, preheat the oven to 400 degrees. Then, slice the tomatoes in half lengthwise.

Place on the baking sheet and drizzle with olive oil. Season it with pepper and salt and then roast in the oven for about 20 minutes. Skins will appear wrinkled when done.

NUTRITION: Calories: 458 Protein: 21 g Fat: 24 g Carbs: 51 g

Greek Yogurt Pancakes

Preparation Time : 10 minutes

Cooking Time: 5 minutes

Servings : 2

INGREDIENTS:

1 cup all-purpose flour

1 cup whole-wheat flour

1/4 teaspoon salt

4 teaspoons baking powder

1 tablespoon sugar

1 1/2 cups unsweetened almond milk

2 teaspoons vanilla extract

2 large eggs

1/2 cup plain 2% Greek yogurt

Fruit, for serving

Maple syrup, for serving

DIRECTIONS:

First, you will have to pour the curds into the bowl and mix them well until creamy. After that, you will have to add egg whites and mix them well until combined.

Then take a separate bowl, pour the wet mixture into the dry mixture. Stir to combine. The batter will be extremely thick.

Then, simply spoon the batter onto the sprayed pan heated too medium-high. The batter must make 4 large pancakes.

Then, you will have to flip the pancakes once when they start to bubble a bit on the surface. Cook until golden brown on both sides.

NUTRITION: Calories: 166 Protein: 14 g Fat: 5 g Carbs: 52g

Mediterranean Feta and Quinoa Egg Muffins

Preparation Time: 15 minutes

Cooking Time : 15 minutes

Servings: 12

INGREDIENTS:

2 cups baby spinach finely chopped

1 cup chopped or sliced cherry tomatoes

1/2 cup finely chopped onion

1 tablespoon chopped fresh oregano

1 cup crumbled feta cheese

1/2 cup chopped {pitted} kalamata olives

2 teaspoons high oleic sunflower oil

1 cup cooked quinoa

8 eggs

1/4 teaspoon salt

DIRECTIONS:

Pre-heat oven to 350 degrees Fahrenheit, and then prepare 12 silicone muffin holders on the baking sheet, or just grease a 12-cup muffin tin with oil and set aside.

Finely chop the vegetables and then heat the skillet to medium. After that, add the vegetable oil and onions and sauté for 2 minutes.

Then, add tomatoes and sauté for another minute, then add spinach and sauté until wilted, about 1 minute.

Place the beaten egg into a bowl and then add lots of vegetables like feta cheese, quinoa, veggie mixture as well as salt, and then stir well until everything is properly combined.

Pour the ready mixture into greased muffin tins or silicone cups, dividing the mixture equally. Then, bake it in an oven for 30 minutes or so.

NUTRITION: Calories: 113 Protein: 6 g Fat: 7 g Carbs: 5 g

Mediterranean Eggs

Preparation Time: 15 minutes

Cooking Time: 20 minutes

Servings: 2

INGREDIENTS:

5 tbsp. of divided olive oil

2 diced medium-sized Spanish onions

2 diced red bell peppers

2 minced cloves garlic

1 teaspoon cumin seeds

4 diced large ripe tomatoes

1 tablespoon of honey

Salt

Freshly ground black pepper

1/3 cup crumbled feta

4 eggs

1 teaspoon zaatar spice

Grilled pita during serving

DIRECTIONS:

Add 3 tablespoons of olive oil into a pan and heat it over medium heat. Along with the oil, sauté the cumin seeds, onions, garlic, and red pepper for a few minutes.

After that, add the diced tomatoes and salt and pepper to taste and cook them for about 10 minutes till they come together and form a light sauce.

With that, half the preparation is already done. Now you just have to break the eggs directly into the sauce and poach them.

However, you must keep in mind to cook the egg whites but keep the yolks still runny. This takes about 8 to 10 minutes.

While plating adds some feta and olive oil with zaatar spice to further enhance the flavors. Once done, serve with grilled pita.

NUTRITION: Calories: 304 Protein: 12 g Fat: 16 g Carbs: 28 g

Pastry-Less Spanakopita

Preparation Time: 5 minutes

Cooking Time: 20 minutes

Servings: 4

INGREDIENTS:

1/8 teaspoons black pepper, add as per taste

1/3 cup of Extra virgin olive oil

4 lightly beaten eggs

7 cups of Lettuce, preferably a spring mix (mesclun)

1/2 cup of crumbled Feta cheese

1/8 teaspoon of Sea salt, add to taste

1 finely chopped medium Yellow onion

DIRECTIONS:

Warm the oven to 180C and grease the flan dish. Once done, pour the extra virgin olive oil into a large saucepan and heat it over medium heat with the onions, until they are translucent.

Add greens and keep stirring until all the ingredients are wilted. Season it with salt and pepper and transfer the greens to the prepared dish and sprinkle on some feta cheese.

Pour the eggs and bake it for 20 minutes till it is cooked through and slightly brown.

NUTRITION: Calories: 325 Protein: 11.2 g Fat: 27.9 g Carbs: 7.3 g

Date and Walnut Overnight Oats

Preparation Time : 5 minutes

Cooking Time: 20 minutes

Servings: 2

INGREDIENTS:

¼ Cup Greek Yogurt, Plain

1/3 cup of yogurt

2/3 cup of oats

1 cup of milk

2 tsp date syrup or you can also use maple syrup or honey

1 mashed banana

¼ tsp cinnamon

¼ cup walnuts

pinch of salt (approx.1/8 tsp)

DIRECTIONS:

Firstly, get a mason jar or a small bowl and add all the ingredients. After that stir and mix all the ingredients well. Cover it securely, and cool it in a refrigerator overnight.

After that, take it out the next morning, add more liquid or cinnamon if required, and serve cold. (However, you can also microwave it for people with a warmer palate.)

NUTRITION: Calories: 350 Protein: 14 g Fat: 12 g Carbs: 49 g

Pear and Mango Smoothie

Preparation time: 5 minutes

Cooking time: 0 minutes

Servings : 1

INGREDIENTS:

   1 ripe mango, cored and chopped
   ½ mango, peeled, pitted and chopped
   1 cup kale, chopped
   ½ cup plain Greek yogurt
   2 ice cubes

DIRECTIONS:

   Add pear, mango, yogurt, kale, and mango to a
      blender and puree. Add ice and blend until you
      have a smooth texture. Serve and enjoy!
NUTRITION: Calories: 293 Fat: 8g Carbohydrates: 53g
Protein: 8g

Eggplant Salad

Preparation time: 20 minutes

Cooking time: 15 minutes

Servings: 8

INGREDIENTS:
- 1 large eggplant, washed and cubed
- 1 tomato, seeded and chopped
- 1 small onion, diced
- 2 tablespoons parsley, chopped
- 2 tablespoons extra virgin olive oil
- 2 tablespoons distilled white vinegar
- ½ cup feta cheese, crumbled
- Salt as needed

DIRECTIONS:
- Pre-heat your outdoor grill to medium-high. Pierce the eggplant a few times using a knife/fork. Cook the eggplants on your grill for about 15 minutes until they are charred.
- Keep it on the side and allow them to cool. Remove the skin from the eggplant and dice the pulp. Transfer the pulp to a mixing bowl and add parsley, onion, tomato, olive oil, feta cheese and vinegar.
- Mix well and chill for 1 hour. Season with salt and enjoy!

NUTRITION: Calories: 99 Fat: 7g Carbohydrates: 7g Protein: 3.4g

Artichoke Frittata

Preparation time: 5 minutes
Cooking time : 10 minutes

Servings : 4

INGREDIENTS:

      8 large eggs
      ¼ cup Asiago cheese, grated
      1 tablespoon fresh basil, chopped
      1 teaspoon fresh oregano, chopped
      Pinch of salt
      1 teaspoon extra virgin olive oil
      1 teaspoon garlic, minced
      1 cup canned artichokes, drained
      1 tomato, chopped

DIRECTIONS:

Pre-heat your oven to broil. Take a medium bowl and whisk in eggs, Asiago cheese, oregano, basil, sea salt and pepper. Blend in a bowl.

Place a large ovenproof skillet over medium-high heat and add olive oil. Add garlic and sauté for 1 minute. Remove skillet from heat and pour in egg mix.

Return skillet to heat and sprinkle artichoke hearts and tomato over eggs. Cook frittata without stirring for 8 minutes.

Place skillet under the broiler for 1 minute until the top is lightly browned. Cut frittata into 4 pieces and serve. Enjoy!

NUTRITION: Calories: 199 Fat: 13g Carbohydrates: 5g Protein: 16g

Full Eggs in a Squash

Preparation time: 15 minutes

Cooking time: 20 minutes

Servings: 5

INGREDIENTS:
- 2 acorn squash
- 6 whole eggs
- 2 tablespoons extra virgin olive oil
- Salt and pepper as needed
- 5-6 pitted dates
- 8 walnut halves
- A fresh bunch of parsley

DIRECTIONS:
- Pre-heat your oven to 375 degrees Fahrenheit. Slice squash crosswise and prepare 3 slices with holes. While slicing the squash, make sure that each slice has a measurement of ¾ inch thickness.
- Remove the seeds from the slices. Take a baking sheet and line it with parchment paper. Transfer the slices to your baking sheet and season them with salt and pepper.
- Bake in your oven for 20 minutes. Chop the walnuts and dates on your cutting board. Take the baking dish out of the oven and drizzle slices with olive oil.
- Crack an egg into each of the holes in the slices and season with pepper and salt. Sprinkle the chopped walnuts on top. Bake for 10 minutes

more. Garnish with parsley and add maple syrup.

NUTRITION: Calories: 198 Fat: 12g Carbohydrates: 17g Protein: 8g

Barley Porridge

Preparation time: 5 minutes

Cooking time: 25 minutes

Servings: 4

INGREDIENTS:
- 1 cup barley
- 1 cup wheat berries
- 2 cups unsweetened almond milk
- 2 cups water
- ½ cup blueberries
- ½ cup pomegranate seeds
- ½ cup hazelnuts, toasted and chopped
- ¼ cup honey

DIRECTIONS:
- Take a medium saucepan and place it over medium-high heat. Place barley, almond milk, wheat berries, water and bring to a boil. Reduce the heat to low and simmer for 25 minutes.
- Divide amongst serving bowls and top each serving with 2 tablespoons blueberries, 2 tablespoons pomegranate seeds, 2 tablespoons hazelnuts, 1 tablespoon honey. Serve and enjoy!

NUTRITION: Calories: 295 Fat: 8g Carbohydrates: 56g Protein: 6g

Tomato and Dill Frittata

Preparation time: 5 minutes

Cooking time: 10 minutes

Servings: 4

INGREDIENTS:

    2 tablespoons olive oil
    1 medium onion, chopped
    1 teaspoon garlic, minced
    2 medium tomatoes, chopped
    6 large eggs
    ½ cup half and half
    ½ cup feta cheese, crumbled
    ¼ cup dill weed
    Salt as needed
    Ground black pepper as needed

DIRECTIONS:

Pre-heat your oven to a temperature of 400 degrees Fahrenheit. Take a large sized ovenproof pan and heat up your olive oil over medium-high heat. Toss in the onion, garlic, tomatoes and stir fry them for 4 minutes.

While they are being cooked, take a bowl and beat together your eggs, half and half cream and season the mix with some pepper and salt.

Pour the mixture into the pan with your vegetables and top it with crumbled feta cheese and dill weed. Cover it with the lid and let it cook for 3 minutes.

Place the pan inside your oven and let it bake for 10 minutes. Serve hot.

NUTRITION: Calories: 191 Fat: 15g Carbohydrates: 6g Protein: 9g

Strawberry and Rhubarb Smoothie

Preparation time: 5 minutes

Cooking time: 3 minutes

Servings: 1

INGREDIENTS:
>1 rhubarb stalk, chopped
>1 cup fresh strawberries, sliced
>½ cup plain Greek strawberries
>Pinch of ground cinnamon
>3 ice cubes

DIRECTIONS:
>Take a small saucepan and fill with water over high heat. Bring to boil and add rhubarb, boil for 3 minutes. Drain and transfer to blender.
>Add strawberries, honey, yogurt, cinnamon and pulse mixture until smooth. Add ice cubes and blend until thick with no lumps. Pour into glass and enjoy chilled.

NUTRITION: Calories: 295 Fat: 8g Carbohydrates: 56g Protein: 6g

Bacon and Brie Omelet Wedges

Preparation time: 10 minutes

Cooking time: 10 minutes

Servings: 6

INGREDIENTS:
- 2 tablespoons olive oil
- 7 ounces smoked bacon
- 6 beaten eggs
- Small bunch chives, snipped
- 3 ½ ounces brie, sliced
- 1 teaspoon red wine vinegar
- 1 teaspoon Dijon mustard
- 1 cucumber, halved, deseeded and sliced diagonally
- 7 ounces radish, quartered

DIRECTIONS:
- Turn your grill on and set it to high. Take a small-sized pan and add 1 teaspoon of oil, allow the oil to heat up. Add lardons and fry until crisp. Drain the lardon on kitchen paper.
- Take another non-sticky cast iron frying pan and place it over grill, heat 2 teaspoons of oil. Add lardons, eggs, chives, ground pepper to the frying pan. Cook on low until they are semi-set.
- Carefully lay brie on top and grill until the Brie sets and is a golden texture. Remove it from the pan and cut up into wedges.

Take a small bowl and create dressing by mixing olive oil, mustard, vinegar and seasoning. Add cucumber to the bowl and mix, serve alongside the omelet wedges.

NUTRITION: Calories: 35 Fat: 31g Carbohydrates: 3g Protein: 25g

Pearl Couscous Salad

Preparation time: 15 minutes

Cooking time: 0 minutes

Servings: 6

INGREDIENTS:

> For Lemon Dill Vinaigrette:
> Juice of 1 large sized lemon
> 1/3 cup of extra virgin olive oil
> 1 teaspoon of dill weed
> 1 teaspoon of garlic powder
> Salt as needed
> Pepper
> For Israeli Couscous:
> 2 cups of Pearl Couscous
> Extra virgin olive oil
> 2 cups of halved grape tomatoes
> Water as needed
> 1/3 cup of finely chopped red onions
> ½ of a finely chopped English cucumber
> 15 ounces of chickpeas
> 14 ounce can of artichoke hearts (roughly chopped up)
> ½ cup of pitted Kalamata olives
> 15-20 pieces of fresh basil leaves, roughly torn and chopped up
> 3 ounces of fresh baby mozzarella

DIRECTIONS:

> Prepare the vinaigrette by taking a bowl and add the ingredients listed under vinaigrette. Mix

them well and keep aside. Take a medium-sized heavy pot and place it over medium heat.

Add 2 tablespoons of olive oil and allow it to heat up. Add couscous and keep cooking until golden brown. Add 3 cups of boiling water and cook the couscous according to the package instructions.

Once done, drain in a colander and keep aside. Take another large-sized mixing bowl and add the remaining ingredients except the cheese and basil.

Add the cooked couscous and basil to the mix and mix everything well. Give the vinaigrette a nice stir and whisk it into the couscous salad. Mix well.

Adjust the seasoning as required. Add mozzarella cheese. Garnish with some basil. Enjoy!

NUTRITION: Calories: 393 Fat: 13g Carbohydrates: 57g Protein: 13g

Coconut Porridge

Preparation time: 15 minutes
Cooking time : 0 minutes

Servings: 6

INGREDIENTS:
>   Powdered erythritol as needed
>   1 ½ cups almond milk, unsweetened
>   2 tablespoons vanilla protein powder
>   3 tablespoons Golden Flaxseed meal
>   2 tablespoons coconut flour

DIRECTIONS:
>   Take a bowl and mix in flaxseed meal, protein powder, coconut flour and mix well. Add mix to saucepan (placed over medium heat).
>   Add almond milk and stir, let the mixture thicken. Add your desired amount of sweetener and serve. Enjoy!

NUTRITION: Calories: 259 Fat: 13g Carbohydrates: 5g Protein: 16g

Crumbled Feta and Scallions

Preparation time: 5 minutes

Cooking time: 15 minutes

Servings: 12

INGREDIENTS:

- 2 tablespoons of unsalted butter (replace with canola oil for full effect)
- ½ cup of chopped up scallions
- 1 cup of crumbled feta cheese
- 8 large sized eggs
- 2/3 cup of milk
- ½ teaspoon of dried Italian seasoning
- Salt as needed
- Freshly ground black pepper as needed
- Cooking oil spray

DIRECTIONS:

Pre-heat your oven to 400 degrees Fahrenheit. Take a 3-4 ounce muffin pan and grease with cooking oil. Take a non-stick pan and place it over medium heat.

Add butter and allow the butter to melt. Add half of the scallions and stir fry. Keep them to the side. Take a medium-sized bowl and add eggs, Italian seasoning and milk and whisk well.

Add the stir fried scallions and feta cheese and mix. Season with pepper and salt. Pour the mix into the muffin tin. Transfer the muffin tin to your oven and bake for 15 minutes. Serve with

a sprinkle of scallions.
NUTRITION: Calories: 106 Fat: 8g Carbohydrates: 2g
Protein: 7g

Quinoa Chicken Salad

Preparation time: 15 minutes

Cooking time: 20 minutes

Servings: 8

INGREDIENTS:
- 2 cups of water
- 2 cubes of chicken bouillon
- 1 smashed garlic clove
- 1 cup of uncooked quinoa
- 2 large sized chicken breasts cut up into bite-sized portions and cooked
- 1 large sized diced red onion
- 1 large sized green bell pepper
- ½ cup of Kalamata olives
- ½ cup of crumbled feta cheese
- ¼ cup of chopped up parsley
- ¼ cup of chopped up fresh chives
- ½ teaspoon of salt
- 1 tablespoon of balsamic vinegar
- ¼ cup of olive oil

DIRECTIONS:

Take a saucepan and bring your water, garlic and bouillon cubes to a boil. Stir in quinoa and reduce the heat to medium low.

Simmer for about 15-20 minutes until the quinoa has absorbed all the water and is tender. Discard your garlic cloves and scrape the quinoa into a large sized bowl.

Gently stir in the cooked chicken breast, bell pepper, onion, feta cheese, chives, salt and parsley into your quinoa.

Drizzle some lemon juice, olive oil and balsamic vinegar. Stir everything until mixed well. Serve warm and enjoy!

NUTRITION: Calories: 99 Fat: 7g Carbohydrates: 7g Protein: 3.4g

Gnocchi Ham Olives

Preparation time : 5 minutes

Cooking time: 15 minutes

Servings: 4

INGREDIENTS:
- 2 tablespoons of olive oil
- 1 medium-sized onion chopped up
- 3 minced cloves of garlic
- 1 medium-sized red pepper completely deseeded and finely chopped
- 1 cup of tomato puree
- 2 tablespoons of tomato paste
- 1 pound of gnocchi
- 1 cup of coarsely chopped turkey ham
- ½ cup of sliced pitted olives
- 1 teaspoon of Italian seasoning
- Salt as needed
- Freshly ground black pepper
- Bunch of fresh basil leaves

DIRECTIONS:
- Take a medium-sized sauce pan and place over medium-high heat. Pour some olive oil and heat it up. Toss in the bell pepper, onion and garlic and sauté for 2 minutes.
- Pour in the tomato puree, gnocchi, tomato paste and add the turkey ham, Italian seasoning and olives. Simmer the whole mix for 15 minutes, making sure to stir from time to time.

Season the mix with some pepper and salt. Once done, transfer the mix to a dish and garnish with some basil leaves. Serve hot and have fun.

NUTRITION: Calories: 335 Fat: 12g Carbohydrates: 45g Protein: 15g

Spicy Early Morning Seafood Risotto

Preparation time: 5 minutes

Cooking time: 15 minutes

Servings: 4

INGREDIENTS:

>3 cups of clam juice
>2 cups of water
>2 tablespoons of olive oil
>1 medium-sized chopped up onion
>2 minced cloves of garlic
>1 ½ cups of Arborio Rice
>½ cup of dry white wine
>1 teaspoon of Saffron
>½ teaspoon of ground cumin
>½ teaspoon of paprika
>1 pound of marinara seafood mix
>Salt as needed
>Ground pepper as needed

DIRECTIONS:

>Place a saucepan over high heat and pour in your clam juice with water and bring the mixture to a boil. Remove the heat.
>Take a heavy bottomed saucepan and stir fry your garlic and onion in oil over medium heat until a nice fragrance comes off.
>Add in the rice and keep stirring for 2-3 minutes until the rice has been fully covered with the oil. Pour the wine and then add the saffron.

Keep stirring constantly until it is fully absorbed. Add in the cumin, clam juice, paprika mixture 1 cup at a time, making sure to keep stirring it from time to time.

Cook the rice for 20 minutes until perfect. Finally, add the seafood marinara mix and cook for another 5-7 minutes.

Season with some pepper and salt. Transfer the meal to a serving dish. Serve hot.

NUTRITION: Calories: 386 Fat: 7g Carbohydrates: 55g Protein: 21g

Rocket Tomatoes and Mushroom Frittata

Preparation time: 5 minutes

Cooking time: 15 minutes

Servings: 4

INGREDIENTS:

- 2 tablespoons of butter (replace with canola oil for full effect)
- 1 chopped up medium-sized onion
- 2 minced cloves of garlic
- 1 cup of coarsely chopped baby rocket tomato
- 1 cup of sliced button mushrooms
- 6 large pieces of eggs
- ½ cup of skim milk
- 1 teaspoon of dried rosemary
- Salt as needed
- Ground black pepper as needed

DIRECTIONS:

Pre-heat your oven to 400 degrees Fahrenheit. Take a large oven-proof pan and place it over medium-heat. Heat up some oil.

Stir fry your garlic, onion for about 2 minutes. Add the mushroom, rosemary and rockets and cook for 3 minutes. Take a medium-sized bowl and beat your eggs alongside the milk.

Season it with some salt and pepper. Pour the egg mixture into your pan with the vegetables and sprinkle some Parmesan.

Reduce the heat to low and cover with the lid. Let it cook for 3 minutes. Transfer the pan into your oven and bake for 10 minutes until fully settled.

Reduce the heat to low and cover with your lid. Let it cook for 3 minutes. Transfer the pan into your oven and then bake for another 10 minutes. Serve hot.

NUTRITION: Calories: 189 Fat: 13g Carbohydrates: 6g Protein: 12g

Cheesy Olives Bread

Preparation Time: 1 hour and 40 minutes

Cooking Time: 30 minutes

Servings: 10

INGREDIENTS:
- 4 cups whole-wheat flour
- 3 tbsps. oregano, chopped
- 2 tsps. dry yeast
- ¼ cup olive oil
- 1 ½ cups black olives, pitted and sliced
- 1 cup of water
- ½ cup feta cheese, crumbled

DIRECTIONS:
- In a bowl, mix the flour with the water, the yeast, and the oil. Stir and knead your dough very well. Put the dough in a bowl, cover with plastic wrap, and keep in a warm place for 1 hour.
- Divide the dough into 2 bowls and stretch each ball well. Add the rest of the ingredients to each ball and tuck them inside. Knead the dough well again.
- Flatten the balls a bit and leave them aside for 40 minutes more. Transfer the balls to a baking sheet lined with parchment paper, make a small slit in each, and bake at 425F for 30 minutes.
- Serve the bread as a Mediterranean breakfast.

NUTRITION: Calories 251 Fat: 7.3g Carbs: 39.7g Protein: 6.7g

Sweet Potato Tart

Preparation Time: 10 minutes
Cooking Time: 1 hour and 10 minutes

Servings: 8

INGREDIENTS:

>2 pounds sweet potatoes, peeled and cubed
>¼ cup olive oil + a drizzle
>7 oz. feta cheese, crumbled
>1 yellow onion, chopped
>2 eggs, whisked
>¼ cup almond milk
>1 tbsp. herbs de Provence
>A pinch of salt and black pepper
>6 phyllo sheets
>1 tbsp. parmesan, grated

DIRECTIONS:

>In a bowl, combine the potatoes with half of the oil, salt, and pepper, toss, spread on a baking sheet lined with parchment paper, and roast at 400F for 25 minutes.

>Meanwhile, heat a pan with half of the remaining oil over medium heat, add the onion, and sauté for 5 minutes.

>In a bowl, combine the eggs with the milk, feta, herbs, salt, pepper, onion, sweet potatoes, and the rest of the oil and toss.

>Arrange the phyllo sheets in a tart pan and brush them with a drizzle of oil. Add the sweet potato mix and spread it well into the pan.

Sprinkle the parmesan on top and bake covered with tin foil at 350F for 20 minutes. Remove the tin foil, bake the tart for 20 minutes more, cool it down, slice, and serve for breakfast.

NUTRITION: Calories 476 Fat: 16.8g Carbs: 68.8g Protein: 13.9g

Stuffed Pita Breads

Preparation Time: 5 minutes

Cooking Time: 15 minutes

Servings: 4

INGREDIENTS:
- 1 ½ tbsp olive oil
- 1 tomato, cubed
- 1 garlic clove, minced
- 1 red onion, chopped
- ¼ cup parsley, chopped
- 15 oz. canned fava beans, drained and rinsed
- ¼ cup lemon juice
- Salt and black pepper to the taste
- 4 whole-wheat pita bread pockets

DIRECTIONS:

Heat a pan with the oil over medium heat, add the onion, stir, and sauté for 5 minutes. Add the rest of the ingredients, stir, and cook for 10 minutes more

Stuff the pita pockets with this mix and serve for breakfast.

NUTRITION: Calories 382 Fat: 1.8g Carbs: 66g Protein: 28.5g

Blueberries Quinoa

Preparation Time: 5 minutes

Cooking Time: 0 minutes

Servings: 4

INGREDIENTS:
>	2 cups almond milk
>	2 cups quinoa, already cooked
>	½ tsp cinnamon powder
>	1 tbsp. honey
>	1 cup blueberries
>	¼ cup walnuts, chopped

DIRECTIONS:
>	In a bowl, mix the quinoa with the milk and the rest of the ingredients, toss, divide into smaller bowls and serve for breakfast.

NUTRITION: Calories 284 Fat: 14.3g Carbs: 15.4g Protein: 4.4g

Endives, Fennel and Orange Salad

Preparation Time: 5 minutes
Cooking Time : 0 minutes

Servings: 4

INGREDIENTS:
- 1 tbsp. balsamic vinegar
- 2 garlic cloves, minced
- 1 tsp. Dijon mustard
- 2 tbsps. olive oil
- 1 tbsp. lemon juice
- Sea salt and black pepper to taste
- ½ cup black olives, pitted and chopped
- 1 tbsp. parsley, chopped
- 7 cups baby spinach
- 2 endives, shredded
- 3 medium navel oranges, peeled and cut into segments
- 2 bulbs fennel, shredded

DIRECTIONS:
In a salad bowl, combine the spinach with the endives, oranges, fennel, and the rest of the ingredients, toss and serve for breakfast.

NUTRITION: Calories 97 Fat: 9.1g Carbs: 3.7g Protein: 1.9g

Raspberries and Yogurt Smoothie

Preparation Time: 5 minutes

Cooking Time: 0 minutes

Servings: 2

INGREDIENTS:

> 2 cups raspberries
> ½ cup Greek yogurt
> ½ cup almond milk
> ½ tsp vanilla extract

DIRECTIONS:

> In your blender, combine the raspberries with the milk, vanilla, and the yogurt, pulse well, divide into 2 glasses and serve for breakfast.

NUTRITION: Calories 245 Fat: 9.5g Carbs: 5.6g Protein: 1.6g

Homemade Muesli

Preparation Time: 15 minutes

Cooking Time: 20 minutes

Servings: 8

INGREDIENTS:
- 3 ½ cups rolled oats
- ½ cup wheat bran
- ½ tsp kosher salt
- ½ tsp ground cinnamon
- ½ cup sliced almonds
- ¼ cup raw pecans, coarsely chopped
- ¼ cup raw pepitas (shelled pumpkin seeds)
- ½ cup unsweetened coconut flakes
- ¼ cup dried apricots, coarsely chopped
- ¼ cup dried cherries

DIRECTIONS:

Take a medium bowl and combine the oats, wheat bran, salt, and cinnamon. Stir well. Place the mixture onto a baking sheet.

Next place the almonds, pecans, and pepitas onto another baking sheet and toss. Pop both trays into the oven and heat to 350°F. Bake for 10-12 minutes. Remove from the oven and pop to one side.

Leave the nuts to cool but take the one with the oats, sprinkle with the coconut, and pop back into the oven for 5 minutes more. Remove and leave to cool. .

Find a large bowl and combine the contents of both trays then stir well to combine. Throw in the apricots and cherries and stir well. Pop into an airtight container until required.

NUTRITION: Calories 250 Fat: 10g Carbs: 36g Protein: 7g

Tangerine and Pomegranate Breakfast Fruit Salad

Preparation Time: 15 minutes

Cooking Time: 20 minutes

Servings: 5

INGREDIENTS:

For the grains:

1 cup pearl or hulled barley

3 cups of water

3 tbsps. olive oil, divided

½ tsp kosher salt

For the fruit:

½ large pineapple, peeled and cut into 1 ½" chunks

6 tangerines

1 ¼ cups pomegranate seeds

1 small bunch of fresh mint

For the dressing:

1/3 cup honey

Juice and finely grated zest of 1 lemon

Juice and finely grated zest of 2 limes

½ tsp kosher salt

¼ cup olive oil

¼ cup toasted hazelnut oil (olive oil is fine too)

DIRECTIONS:

Place the grain into a strainer and rinse well. Grab 2 baking sheets, line with paper, and add the grain. Spread well to cover then leave to dry.

Next, place the water into a saucepan and pop over medium heat. Place a skillet over medium heat, add 2 tbsps. of the oil then add the barley. Toast for 2 minutes.

Add the water and salt and bring to a boil. Reduce to simmer and cook for 40 minutes until most of the liquid has been absorbed. Turn off the heat and leave to stand for 10 minutes to steam cook the rest.

Meanwhile, grab a medium bowl and add the honey, juices, zest, and salt, and stir well. Add the olive oil then nut oil and stir again. Pop until the fridge until needed.

Remove the lid from the barley then place it onto another prepared baking sheet and leave to cool. Drizzle with oil and leave to cool completely then pop into the fridge.

When ready to serve, divide the grains, pineapple, orange, pomegranate, and mint between the bowls. Drizzle with the dressing then serve and enjoy.

NUTRITION: Calories 400 Fat: 23g Carbs: 50g Protein: 3g

Hummus and Tomato Breakfast Pittas

Preparation Time: 5 minutes

Cooking Time: 10 minutes

Servings: 4

INGREDIENTS:
- 4 large eggs, at room temperature
- Salt, to taste
- 2 whole-wheat pita bread with pockets, cut in half
- ½cup hummus
- 1 medium cucumber, thinly sliced into rounds
- 2 medium tomatoes, large dice
- A handful of fresh parsley leaves, coarsely chopped
- Freshly ground black pepper
- Hot sauce (optional)

DIRECTIONS:
- Grab a large saucepan, fill with water, and pop over medium heat until it boils. Add the eggs and cook for 7 minutes.
- Immediately drain the water and place the eggs under cool water until they cool down. Pop to one side until you can handle them comfortably.
- Peel the eggs and cut them into ¼" slices, sprinkle with salt, and pop to one side.
- Grab a pitta pocket and spread with hummus, fill with cucumber and tomato, season well then add an egg. Sprinkle with parsley and hot

sauce then serve and enjoy.
NUTRITION: Calories 377 Fat: 31g Carbs: 17g Protein: 11g

Baked Ricotta & Pears

Preparation Time: 15 minutes
Cooking Time : 30 minutes

Servings: 4

INGREDIENTS:
- ¼ cup White whole wheat flour
- 1 tbsp. Sugar
- ¼ tsp Nutmeg
- Ricotta cheese
- 16 oz. container whole-milk
- 2Large eggs
- 1Diced pear
- 2 tbsp. Water
- 1 tsp. Vanilla extract
- 1 tbsp. Honey
- Also Needed: 4 - 6 oz. ramekins

DIRECTIONS:
Warm the oven to 400°F. Lightly spritz the ramekins with a cooking oil spray. Whisk the flour, nutmeg, sugar, vanilla, eggs, and ricotta together in a large mixing container.

Spoon the fixings into the dishes. Bake them for 20 to 25 minutes or until they're firm and set. Transfer them to the countertop and wait for them to cool.

In a saucepan, using the medium temperature setting, toss the cored and diced pear into the water for about ten minutes until it's slightly softened.

Take the pan from the burner and stir in the honey. Serve the ricotta ramekins with the warm pear when it's ready.

NUTRITION: Calories 312 Protein: 17g Carbs: 0g Fat: 17g

Shakshuka With Feta

Preparation time : 15 minutes

Cooking time: 41 minutes

Servings: 4-6

INGREDIENTS:

>6 large eggs
>3 tbsp extra-virgin olive oil
>1 large onion, halved and thinly sliced
>1 large red bell pepper, seeded and thinly sliced
>3 garlic cloves, thinly sliced
>1 tsp ground cumin
>1 tsp sweet paprika
>1/8 tsp cayenne, or to taste
>1 (28-ounce) can whole plum tomatoes with juices, coarsely chopped
>¾ tsp salt, more as needed
>¼ tsp black pepper, more as needed
>5 oz feta cheese, crumbled, about 1 1/4 cups
>To Serve:
>Chopped cilantro
>Hot sauce

DIRECTIONS:

>Preheat oven to 375 degrees F. In a large skillet over medium-low heat, add the oil. Once heated, add the onion and bell pepper, cook gently until very soft, about 20 minutes.
>Add in the garlic and cook until tender, 1 to 2 minutes, then stir in cumin, paprika and cayenne, and cook 1 minute.

Pour in tomatoes, season with 3/4 tsp salt and 1/4 tsp pepper, simmer until tomatoes have thickened, about 10 minutes. Then stir in crumbled feta.

Gently crack eggs into skillet over tomatoes, season with salt and pepper. Transfer skillet to oven. Bake until eggs have just set, 7 to 10 minutes. Serve.

NUTRITION: Calories: 337 Carbs: 17g Fat: 25g Protein: 12g

Peanut Butter Banana Greek Yogurt

Preparation time: 15 minutes
Cooking time   : 0 minutes

Servings: 4

INGREDIENTS:

       3 cups vanilla Greek yogurt
       2 medium bananas sliced
       1/4 cup creamy natural peanut butter
       1/4 cup flaxseed meal
       1 tsp nutmeg

DIRECTIONS:

Divide yogurt between four jars with lids. Top with banana slices.

In a bowl, melt the peanut butter in a microwave safe bowl for 30-40 seconds and drizzle one tbsp on each bowl on top of the bananas. Store in the fridge for up to 3 days.

When ready to serve, sprinkle with flaxseed meal and ground nutmeg. Enjoy!

NUTRITION: Calories: 370 Carbs: 47g Fat: 10g Protein: 22g

Veggie Mediterranean Quiche

Preparation time: 15 minutes
Cooking time : 55 minutes

Servings: 8

INGREDIENTS:

  1/2 cup sundried tomatoes - dry or in olive oil
  Boiling water
  1 prepared pie crust
  2 tbsp vegan butter
  1 onion, diced
  2 cloves garlic, minced
  1 red pepper, diced
  1/4 cup sliced Kalamata olives
  1 tsp dried oregano
  1 tsp dried parsley
  1/3 cup crumbled feta cheese
  4 large eggs
  1 1/4 cup milk
  2 cups fresh spinach or 1/2 cup frozen spinach, thawed and squeezed dry
  Salt, to taste
  Pepper, to taste
  1 cup shredded cheddar cheese, divided

DIRECTIONS:

  If you're using dry sundried tomatoes - In a measure cup, add the sundried tomatoes and pour the boiling water over until just covered, allow to sit for 5 minutes or until the tomatoes are soft. The drain and chop tomatoes, set aside.

Preheat oven to 375 degrees F. Fit a 9-inch pie plate with the prepared pie crust, then flute edges, and set aside. In a skillet over medium high heat, melt the butter.

Add in the onion and garlic, and cook until fragrant and tender, about 3 minutes. Add in the red pepper, cook for an additional 3 minutes, or until the peppers are just tender.

Add in the spinach, olives, oregano, and parsley, cook until the spinach is wilted (if you're using fresh) or heated through (if you're using frozen), about 5 minutes.

Remove the pan from heat, stir in the feta cheese and tomatoes, spoon the mixture into the prepared pie crust, spreading out evenly, set aside.

In a medium-sized mixing bowl, whisk together the eggs, 1/2 cup of the cheddar cheese, milk, salt, and pepper. Pour this egg and cheese mixture evenly over the spinach mixture in the pie crust.

Sprinkle top with the remaining cheddar cheese. Bake for 50-55 minutes, or until the crust is golden brown and the egg is set. Allow to cool completely before slicing.

NUTRITION: Calories: 239 Carbs: 19g Fat: 15g Protein: 7g

Spinach, Feta and Egg Breakfast Quesadillas

Preparation time: 15 minutes

Cooking time: 15 minutes

Servings: 5

INGREDIENTS:

 8 eggs (optional)
 2 tsp olive oil
 1 red bell pepper
 1/2 red onion
 1/4 cup milk
 4 handfuls of spinach leaves
 1 1/2 cup mozzarella cheese
 5 sun-dried tomato tortillas
 1/2 cup feta
 1/4 tsp salt
 1/4 tsp pepper
 Spray oil

DIRECTIONS:

 In a large non-stick pan over medium heat, add the olive oil. Once heated, add the bell pepper and onion, cook for 4-5 minutes until soft.

 In the meantime, whisk together the eggs, milk, salt and pepper in a bowl. Add in the egg/milk mixture into the pan with peppers and onions, stirring frequently, until eggs are almost cooked through.

 Add in the spinach and feta, fold into the eggs, stirring until spinach is wilted and eggs are cooked through. Remove the eggs from heat and plate.

Spray a separate large non-stick pan with spray oil, and place over medium heat. Add the tortilla, on one half of the tortilla, spread about ½ cup of the egg mixture.

Top the eggs with around 1/3 cup of shredded mozzarella cheese. Fold the second half of the tortilla over, then cook for 2 minutes, or until golden brown.

Flip and cook for another minute until golden brown. Allow the quesadilla to cool completely, divide among the container, store for 2 days or wrap in plastic wrap and foil, and freeze for up to 2 months

NUTRITION: Calories: 213 Fat: 11g Carbs: 15g Protein: 15g

Mediterranean Quinoa and Feta Egg Muffins

Preparation time: 15 minutes

Cooking time: 30 minutes

Servings: 12

INGREDIENTS:
- 8 eggs
- 1 cup cooked quinoa
- 1 cup crumbled feta cheese
- 1/4 tsp salt
- 2 cups baby spinach finely chopped
- 1/2 cup finely chopped onion
- 1 cup chopped or sliced tomatoes, cherry or grape tomatoes
- 1/2 cup chopped and pitted Kalamata olives
- 1 tbsp chopped fresh oregano
- 2 tsp high oleic sunflower oil plus optional extra for greasing muffin tins

DIRECTIONS:
Pre-heat oven to 350 degrees F. Prepare 12 silicone muffin holders on a baking sheet, or grease a 12-cup muffin tin with oil, set aside.

In a skillet over medium heat, add the vegetable oil and onions, sauté for 2 minutes. Add tomatoes, sauté for another minute, then add spinach and sauté until wilted, about 1 minute.

Remove from heat and stir in olives and oregano, set aside. Place the eggs in a blender or mixing bowl and blend or mix until well combined.

Pour the eggs in to a mixing bowl (if you used a blender) then add quinoa, feta cheese, veggie mixture, and salt, and stir until well combined.

Pour mixture in to silicone cups or greased muffin tins, dividing equally, and bake for 30 minutes, or until eggs have set and muffins are a light golden brown. Allow to cool completely.

NUTRITION: Calories: 113 Carbohydrates: 5g Fat: 7g Protein: 6g

Green Shakshuka

Preparation time: 15 minutes

Cooking time: 15 minutes

Servings: 2

INGREDIENTS:

    1 tbsp olive oil
    1 onion, peeled and diced
    1 clove garlic, peeled and finely minced
    3 cups broccoli rabe, chopped
    3 cups baby spinach leaves
    2 tbsp whole milk or cream
    1 tsp ground cumin
    1/4 tsp black pepper
    1/4 tsp salt (or to taste)
    4 Eggs
    Garnish:
    1 pinch sea salt
    1 pinch red pepper flakes

DIRECTIONS:

    Pre-heat the oven to 350 degrees F. Add the broccoli rabe to a large pot of boiling water, cook for 2 minutes, drain and set aside.

    In a large oven-proof skillet or cast-iron pan over medium heat, add in the tablespoon of olive oil along with the diced onions, cook for about 10 minutes or until the onions become translucent.

    Add the minced garlic and continue cooking for about another minute. Cut the par-cooked broccoli rabe into small pieces, stir into the onion and garlic mixture.

Cook for a couple of minutes, then stir in the baby spinach leaves, continue to cook for a couple more minutes, stirring often, until the spinach begins to wilt. Stir in the ground cumin, salt, ground black pepper, and milk.

Make four wells in the mixture, crack an egg into each well – be careful not to break the yolks. Also, note that it's easier to crack each egg into a small bowl and then transfer them to the pan.

Place the pan with the eggs into the pre-heated oven, cook for 10 to 15 minutes until the eggs are set to preference. Sprinkle the cooked eggs with a dash of sea salt and a pinch of red pepper flakes.

NUTRITION: Calories: 278 Carbs: 18g Fat: 16g Protein: 16g

Apple Quinoa Breakfast Bars

Preparation time: 15 minutes
Cooking time : 40 minutes

Servings: 12

INGREDIENTS:
>   2 eggs
>   1 apple peeled and chopped into ½ inch chunks
>   1 cup unsweetened apple sauce
>   1 ½ cups cooked & cooled quinoa
>   1 ½ cups rolled oats
>   1/4 cup peanut butter
>   1 tsp vanilla
>   1/2 tsp cinnamon
>   1/4 cup coconut oil
>   ½ tsp baking powder

DIRECTIONS:
>   Heat oven to 350 degrees F. Spray an 8x8 inch baking dish with oil, set aside. In a large bowl, stir together the apple sauce, cinnamon, coconut oil, peanut butter, vanilla and eggs.
>   Add in the cooked quinoa, rolled oats and baking powder, mix until completely incorporated. Fold in the apple chunks.
>   Spread the mixture into the prepared baking dish, spreading it to each corner. Bake for 40 minutes, or until a toothpick comes out clean. Allow to cool before slicing.

NUTRITION: Calories: 230 Fat: 10g Carbs: 31g Protein: 7g

Mediterranean Breakfast Salad

Preparation time: 15 minutes

Cooking time: 10 minutes

Servings: 2

INGREDIENTS:
- 4 eggs (optional)
- 10 cups arugula
- 1/2 seedless cucumber, chopped
- 1 cup cooked quinoa, cooled
- 1 large avocado
- 1 cup natural almonds, chopped
- 1/2 cup mixed herbs like mint and dill, chopped
- 2 cups halved cherry tomatoes and/or heirloom tomatoes cut into wedges
- Extra virgin olive oil
- 1 lemon
- Sea salt, to taste
- Freshly ground black pepper, to taste

DIRECTIONS:
- Cook the eggs by soft-boiling them - Bring a pot of water to a boil, then reduce heat to a simmer. Gently lower all the eggs into water and allow them to simmer for 6 minutes.
- Remove the eggs from water and run cold water on top to stop the cooking, process set aside and peel when ready to use.
- In a large bowl, combine the arugula, tomatoes, cucumber, and quinoa. Divide the salad among

2 containers, store in the fridge for 2 days.
NUTRITION: Calories: 252 Carbs: 18g Fat: 16g Protein: 10g

Greek Quinoa Breakfast Bowl

Preparation time: 15 minutes
Cooking time : 20 minutes

Servings: 6

INGREDIENTS:

  12 eggs
  ¼ cup plain Greek yogurt
  1 tsp onion powder
  1 tsp granulated garlic
  ½ tsp salt
  ½ tsp pepper
  1 tsp olive oil
  1 (5 oz) bag baby spinach
  1 pint cherry tomatoes, halved
  1 cup feta cheese
  2 cups cooked quinoa

DIRECTIONS:

  In a large bowl whisk together eggs, Greek yogurt, onion powder, granulated garlic, salt, and pepper, set aside.

  In a large skillet, heat olive oil and add spinach, cook the spinach until it is slightly wilted, about 3-4 minutes.

  Add in cherry tomatoes, cook until tomatoes are softened, 3-4 minutes. Stir in egg mixture and cook until the eggs are set, about 7-9 minutes, stir in the eggs as they cook to scramble.

Once the eggs have set stir in the feta and quinoa, cook until heated through. Distribute evenly among the containers, store for 2-3 days.
NUTRITION: Calories: 357 Carbohydrates: 8g Fat: 20g Protein: 23g

Mushroom Goat Cheese Frittata

Preparation time: 15 minutes

Cooking time: 35 minutes

Servings: 4

INGREDIENTS:

     1 tbsp olive oil
     1 small onion, diced
     10 oz cremini or your favorite mushrooms, sliced
     1 garlic clove, minced
     10 eggs
     2/3 cup half and half
     1/4 cup fresh chives, minced
     2 tsp fresh thyme, minced
     1/2 tsp kosher salt
     1/2 tsp black pepper
     4 oz goat cheese

DIRECTIONS:

Preheat the oven to 375 degrees F. In an over safe skillet or cast-iron pan over medium heat, olive oil. Add in the onion and sauté for 3-5 mins until golden.

Add in the sliced mushrooms and garlic, continue to sauté until mushrooms are golden brown, about 10-12 minutes.

In a large bowl, whisk together the eggs, half and half, chives, thyme, salt and pepper. Place the goat cheese over the mushroom mixture and pour the egg mixture over the top.

Stir the MIXTURE in the pan and cook over medium heat until the edges are set but the center is still loose, about 8-10 minutes

Put the pan in the oven and finish cooking for an additional 8-10 minutes or until set. Allow to cool completely before slicing.

NUTRITION: Calories: 243 Carbohydrates: 5g Fat: 17g Protein: 15g

Mediterranean Frittata

Preparation Time: 8 minutes

Cooking Time: 6 minutes

Servings: 4

INGREDIENTS:

> 2 teaspoons of olive oil
> 3/4 cup of baby spinach, packed
> 2 green onions
> 4 egg whites, large
> 6 large eggs
> 1/3 cup of crumbled feta cheese, (1.3 ounces) along with sun-dried tomatoes and basil
> 2 teaspoons of salt-free Greek seasoning
> 1/4 teaspoon of salt

DIRECTIONS:

> Take a boiler and preheat it. Take a ten-inch ovenproof skillet and pour the oil into it and keep the skillet on a medium flame.
> While the oil gets heated, chop the spinach roughly and the onions. Put the eggs, egg whites, Greek seasoning, cheese, as well as salt in a large mixing bowl and mix it thoroughly using a whisker.
> Add the chopped spinach and onions into the mixing bowl and stir it well.
> Pour the mixture into the pan and cook it for 2 minutes or more until the edges of the mixture set well.

Lift the edges of the mixture gently and tilt the pan so that the uncooked portion can get underneath it. Cook for another two minutes so that the whole mixture gets cooked properly.

Broil for two to three minutes till the center gets set. Your Frittata is now ready. Serve it hot by cutting it into four wedges.

NUTRITION: Calories: 178 Protein: 16 g Fat: 12 g Carbs: 2.2 g

Honey-Caramelized Figs with Greek Yogurt

Preparation Time: 5 minutes
Cooking Time : 5 minutes

Servings: 4

INGREDIENTS:

>   4 fresh halved figs
>   2 tablespoons of melted butter, 30ml
>   2 tablespoons of brown sugar, 30ml
>   2 cups of Greek yogurt 500ml
>   1/4 cup of honey, 60ml

DIRECTIONS:

>   Take a non-stick skillet and preheat it over a medium flame. Put the butter on the pan and toss the figs into it and sprinkle in some brown sugar over it.
>   Put the figs on the pan and cut off the side of the figs. Cook the figs on a medium flame for 2-3 minutes until they turn a golden brown.
>   Turn over the figs and cook them for 2-3 minutes again. Remove the figs from the pan and let it cool down a little.
>   Take a plate and put a scoop of Greek yogurt on it. Put the cooked figs over the yogurts and drizzle the honey over it

NUTRITION: Calories: 350 Protein: 6 g Fat: 19 g Carbs: 40 g

Savory Quinoa Egg Muffins with Spinach

Preparation Time: 15 minutes

Cooking Time: 20 minutes

Servings: 2

INGREDIENTS:
- 1 cup of quinoa
- 2 cups of water/ vegetable broth)
- 4 ounces of spinach which is about one cup
- 1/2 chopped onion
- 2 whole eggs
- 1/4 cup of grated cheese
- 1/2 teaspoon of oregano or thyme
- 1/2 teaspoon of garlic powder
- 1/2 teaspoon of salt

DIRECTIONS:
- Take a medium saucepan and put water in it. Add the quinoa in the water and bring the whole thing to a simmer.
- Cover the pan and cook it for 10 minutes till the water gets absorbed by the quinoa. Remove the saucepan from the heat and let it cool down.
- Take a nonstick pan and heat the onions till they turn soft and then add spinach. Cook all of them together till the spinach gets a little wilted and then remove it from the heat.
- Preheat the oven to 176 C. Take a muffin pan and grease it lightly.

Take a large bowl and add the cooked quinoa along with the cooked onions, spinach, and add cheese, eggs, thyme or oregano, salt, garlic powder, pepper and mix them together.

Put a spoonful of the mixture into a muffin tin. Make sure it is ¼ of a cup. In the preheated pan, put it in the pan and bake it for around 20 minutes.

NUTRITION: Calories: 61 Protein: 4 g Fat: 3 g Carbs: 6 g

Avocado Tomato Gouda Socca Pizza

Preparation Time: 20 minutes

Cooking Time: 20 minutes

Servings: 2

INGREDIENTS:
- 1 and 1/4 cups of chickpea or garbanzo bean flour
- 1 and 1/4 cups of cold water
- 1/4 teaspoon of pepper and sea salt each
- 2 teaspoons of avocado or olive oil + 1 teaspoon extra for heating the pan
- 1 teaspoon of minced Garlic which will be around two cloves
- 1 teaspoon of Onion powder/other herb seasoning powder
- 10 to twelve-inch cast iron pan
- 1 sliced tomato
- 1/2 avocado
- 2 ounces of thinly sliced Gouda
- 1/4-1/3 cup of Tomato sauce
- 2 or 3 teaspoons of chopped green scallion/onion
- Sprouted greens for green
- Extra pepper/salt for sprinkling on top of the pizza
- Red pepper flakes

DIRECTIONS:
Mix the flour with two teaspoons of olive oil, herbs, water, and whisk it until a smooth mixture form. Keep it at room temperature for around 15-20 minutes to let the batter settle.

In the meantime, preheat the oven and place the pan inside the oven and let it get heated for around 10 minutes. When the pan gets preheated, chop up the vegetables into fine slices.

Remove the pan after ten minutes using oven mitts. Put one teaspoon of oil and swirl it all around to coat the pan.

Pour the batter into the pan and tilt the pan so that the batter spreads evenly throughout the pan. Turn down the over to 425f and place back the pan for 5-8 minutes.

Remove the pan from the oven and add the sliced avocado, tomato and on top of that, add the gouda slices and the onion slices.

Put the pizza back into the oven and wait till the cheese get melted or the sides of the bread gets crusty and brown.

Remove the pizza from the pan and add the microgreens on top, along with the toppings.

NUTRITION: Calories: 416 Protein: 15 g Fat: 10 g Carbs: 37 g

Sunny-Side Up Baked Eggs with Swiss Chard, Feta, and Basil

Preparation Time: 15 minutes

Cooking Time: 10 minutes

Servings: 4

INGREDIENTS:
- 4 bell peppers, any color
- 1 tablespoon extra-virgin olive oil
- 8 large eggs
- ¾ teaspoon kosher salt, divided
- ¼ teaspoon freshly ground black pepper, divided
- 1 avocado, peeled, pitted, and diced
- ¼ cup red onion, diced
- ¼ cup fresh basil, chopped
- Juice of ½ lime

DIRECTIONS:
- Stem and seed the bell peppers. Cut 2 (2-inch-thick) rings from each pepper. Chop the remaining bell pepper into small dice and set aside.
- Heat the olive oil in a large skillet over medium heat. Add 4 bell pepper rings, then crack 1 egg in the middle of each ring.
- Season with ¼ teaspoon of the salt and 1/8 teaspoon of the black pepper. Cook until the egg whites are mostly set, but the yolks are still runny 2 to 3 minutes.

Gently flip and cook 1 additional minute for over easy. Move the egg–bell pepper rings to a platter or onto plates and repeats with the remaining 4 bell pepper rings.

In a medium bowl, combine the avocado, onion, basil, lime juice, reserved diced bell pepper, the remaining ¼ teaspoon kosher salt, and the remaining 1/8 teaspoon black pepper. Divide among the 4 plates.

NUTRITION: Calories: 270 Protein: 15 g Fat: 19 g Carbs: 12 g

Polenta with Sautéed Chard and Fried Eggs

Preparation Time: 5 minutes

Cooking Time: 20 minutes

Servings: 4

INGREDIENTS:
- 2½ cups water
- ½ teaspoon kosher salt
- ¾ cups whole-grain cornmeal
- ¼ teaspoon freshly ground black pepper
- 2 tablespoons grated Parmesan cheese
- 1 tablespoon extra-virgin olive oil
- 1 bunch (about 6 ounces) Swiss chard, leaves and stems chopped and separated
- 2 garlic cloves, sliced
- ¼ teaspoon kosher salt
- 1/8 teaspoon freshly ground black pepper
- Lemon juice (optional)
- 1 tablespoon extra-virgin olive oil
- 4 large eggs

DIRECTIONS:
For the polenta, bring the water and salt to a boil in a medium saucepan over high heat. Slowly add the cornmeal, whisking constantly.

Decrease the heat to low, cover, and cook for 10 to 15 minutes, stirring often to avoid lumps. Stir in the pepper and Parmesan and divide among 4 bowls.

For the chard, heat the oil in a large skillet over medium heat. Add the chard stems, garlic, salt, and pepper; sauté for 2 minutes. Add the chard leaves and cook until wilted, about 3 to 5 minutes.

Add a spritz of lemon juice (if desired), toss together, and divide evenly on top of the polenta.

For the eggs, heat the oil in the same large skillet over medium-high heat. Crack each egg into the skillet, taking care not to crowd the skillet and leaving space between the eggs.

Cook until the whites are set and golden around the edges, about 2 to 3 minutes. Serve sunny-side up or flip the eggs over carefully and cook 1 minute longer for over easy. Place one egg on top of the polenta and chard in each bowl.

NUTRITION: Calories: 310 Protein: 17 g Fat: 18 g Carbs: 21 g

Smoked Salmon Egg Scramble with Dill and Chives

Preparation Time: 5 minutes
Cooking Time : 5 minutes

Servings: 2

INGREDIENTS:
- 4 large eggs
- 1 tablespoon milk
- 1 tablespoon fresh chives, minced
- 1 tablespoon fresh dill, minced
- ¼ teaspoon kosher salt
- 1/8 teaspoon freshly ground black pepper
- 2 teaspoons extra-virgin olive oil
- 2 ounces smoked salmon, thinly sliced

DIRECTIONS:
In a large bowl, whisk together the eggs, milk, chives, dill, salt, and pepper. Heat the olive oil in a medium skillet or sauté pan over medium heat.

Add the egg mixture and cook for about 3 minutes, stirring occasionally. Add the salmon and cook until the eggs are set but moist about 1 minute.

NUTRITION: Calories: 325 Protein: 23 g Fat: 26 g Carbs: 1 g

Eggs with Zucchini Noodles

Preparation Time: 10 minutes

Cooking Time: 11 minutes

Servings: 2

INGREDIENTS:

    2 tablespoons extra-virgin olive oil
    3 zucchinis, cut with a spiralizer
    4 eggs
    Salt and black pepper to the taste
    A pinch of red pepper flakes
    Cooking spray
    1 tablespoon basil, chopped

DIRECTIONS:

    In a bowl, combine the zucchini noodles with salt, pepper, and the olive oil, and toss well. Grease a baking sheet with cooking spray and divide the zucchini noodles into 4 nests on it.

    Crack an egg on top of each nest, sprinkle salt, pepper, and the pepper flakes on top, and bake at 350 degrees F for 11 minutes. Divide the mix between plates, sprinkle the basil on top, and serve.

NUTRITION: Calories: 296 Protein: 15 g Fat: 24 g Carbs: 11 g

Banana Oats

Preparation Time: 10 minutes
Cooking Time : 0 minutes

Servings: 2

INGREDIENTS:

- 1 banana, peeled and sliced
- ¾ cup almond milk
- ½ cup cold-brewed coffee
- 2 dates, pitted
- 2 tablespoons cocoa powder
- 1 cup rolled oats
- 1 and ½ tablespoons chia seeds

DIRECTIONS:

In a blender, combine the banana with the milk and the rest of the ingredients, pulse, divide into bowls and serve for breakfast.

NUTRITION: Calories: 451 Protein: 9 g Fat: 25 g Carbs: 55 g

Slow-Cooked Peppers Frittata

Preparation Time: 10 minutes

Cooking Time: 3 hours

Servings: 6

INGREDIENTS:
- ½ cup almond milk
- 8 eggs, whisked
- Salt and black pepper to the taste
- 1 teaspoon oregano, dried
- 1 and ½ cups roasted peppers, chopped
- ½ cup red onion, chopped
- 4 cups baby arugula
- 1 cup goat cheese, crumbled
- Cooking spray

DIRECTIONS:

In a bowl, combine the eggs with salt, pepper, and the oregano and whisk. Grease your slow cooker with the cooking spray, arrange the peppers and the remaining ingredients inside and pour the egg mixture over them.

Put the lid on and cook on Low for 3 hours. Divide the frittata between plates and serve.

NUTRITION: Calories: 259 Protein: 16 g Fat: 20 g Carbs: 4.4 g

Slow Cooked Turkey and Brown Rice

Preparation time: 15 minutes
Cooking time: 3 hours & 10 minutes

Servings: 6

INGREDIENTS:

>   1 tablespoon extra-virgin olive oil
>   1½ pounds (680 g) ground turkey
>   2 tablespoons chopped fresh sage, divided
>   2 tablespoons chopped fresh thyme, divided
>   1 teaspoon sea salt
>   ½ teaspoon ground black pepper
>   2 cups brown rice
>   1 (14-ounce / 397-g) can stewed tomatoes, with the juice
>   ¼ cup pitted and sliced Kalamata olives
>   3 medium zucchinis, sliced thinly
>   ¼ cup chopped fresh flat-leaf parsley
>   1 medium yellow onion, chopped
>   1 tablespoon plus 1 teaspoon balsamic vinegar
>   2 cups low-sodium chicken stock
>   2 garlic cloves, minced
>   ½ cup grated Parmesan cheese, for serving

DIRECTIONS:

>   Heat the olive oil in a nonstick skillet over medium-high heat until shimmering. Add the ground turkey and sprinkle with 1 tablespoon of sage, 1 tablespoon of thyme, salt and ground black pepper.

Sauté for 10 minutes or until the ground turkey is lightly browned. Pour them in the slow cooker, then pour in the remaining ingredients, except for the Parmesan. Stir to mix well.

Put the lid on and cook on high for 3 hours or until the rice and vegetables are tender. Pour them in a large serving bowl, then spread with Parmesan cheese before serving.

NUTRITION: Calories: 499 Fat: 16.4g Protein: 32.4g Carbs: 56.5g